RED CROSS FIRST AID MODULE

CPR:
Race for Life

A: Airway tip head check fr breathing

If No breathing

Quick: 4 Quick Breaths

Check: ✓ pulse & breathing

15 comp 2 breaths
15 ,,   2 ,,
15 ,,   2
15 ,,   2
_____
✓ pulse & breathing

ISBN: 0-86536-024-3

PREFACE

The Red Cross Modular System is organized into units so that the content of courses of instruction can be tailored to the needs of different student groups. This module teaches emergency first aid for respiratory failure and cardiac arrest in adult victims. Topics include mouth-to-mouth breathing and one-rescuer cardiopulmonary resuscitation (CPR). In view of the large number of cardiac emergencies that occur each year, we urge all students of first aid to become certified in CPR.

Modules are designed to be used either entirely in a classroom setting or for home study and practice, with later practice, testing, and checkout of skills being carried out in the classroom under supervision of a Red Cross instructor. Your instructor will tell you how to schedule your work in this course.

This book is self-instructional. Answer the questions in the book, then check your answers on the pages following the questions. In each unit there is a practice session that you will do with one or more other students. Your instructor will check your performance in each practice session. Manikins are recommended for practice and checkout of mouth-to-mouth breathing, and they are required for CPR.

ACKNOWLEDGMENTS

The content of <u>CPR: Race for Life</u> is based on information provided by the Division of Medical Sciences, National Academy of Sciences, National Research Council (NAS, NRC). The American Heart Association cooperated in setting compatible technical standards for AHA and Red Cross materials. This edition reflects the updating of standards recommended by the 1979 National Conference on Cardiopulmonary Resuscitation and Emergency Cardiac Care.

The Red Cross thanks Sam F. Seeley, M.D., who gave technical guidance for preparation of the American Red Cross <u>Advanced First Aid and Emergency Care</u> textbook before his retirement as Professional Associate for the Division of Medical Sciences of NAS, NRC. Dr. Seeley's continued interest and assistance after his retirement are greatly valued by the Red Cross. The Red Cross also gives special thanks to Archer S. Gordon, M.D., Ph.D., for technical guidance and advice in developing these materials on respiratory and circulatory emergencies.

The instructional research and development of this module were carried out by Communication Research Laboratories, Inc., Steamboat Springs, Colorado, under the supervision of David G. Markle, Ph.D. and Nancy H. Markle, Ph.D., Co-Directors. Roseanna L. Dufault, Kathy M. Dietrich, and Patsy L. Parkin were Project Assistants; illustrations are by Monica King and Scott Gorrell.

Review and guidance for technical consistency were provided by C. P. Dail, Jr., Director of First Aid Programs, American Red Cross, and Don A. Sleeper, Assistant Director of First Aid Programs, American Red Cross.

Thanks are extended to the following Red Cross chapters for assistance in testing these materials: Alexandria Chapter, Alexandria, Va.; Berkeley Chapter, Berkeley, Calif.; Central Pennsylvania Division, Harrisburg Chapter, Harrisburg, Pa.; Goddard Space Flight Center, Greenbelt, Md.; Laurel Parks and Recreation Department, Laurel, Md.; Prince George's County Chapter, Hyattsville, Md.; San Diego County Chapter, San Diego, Calif.; and Seattle-King County Chapter, Seattle, Wash.

The Red Cross Modular System is dedicated to the thousands of volunteers who give their time and abilities to provide lifesaving information to the American public.

EMERGENCY MEDICAL SERVICES (EMS) SYSTEM

An EMS system is a community-wide, coordinated means of responding to an accident or sudden illness. You should know about these three features of an EMS system: (1) entry into the system, (2) rescue and transportation, and (3) hospital emergency facilities.

<u>Entry into the System</u>. Two kinds of action are needed to enter a victim into the EMS system:

Action 1: Bystanders provide immediate emergency care, which greatly increases the survival chances of a victim of an accident or sudden illness. As many people as possible should be trained in first aid and CPR.

Action 2: At the same time or as soon as possible, another bystander "activates the EMS system." Telephone 911 or 0 or the local EMS number (see inside front cover of phone directory). There is space for emergency numbers on the back cover of this book. When you call for help, tell:

1. <u>WHERE</u> the emergency situation is, with cross streets if possible.
2. <u>PHONE NUMBER</u> you are calling from.
3. <u>WHAT HAPPENED</u>—heart attack, auto accident, fall, etc.
4. <u>HOW MANY</u> persons need help.
5. <u>WHAT is being done</u> for the victims.
6. <u>YOU HANG UP LAST</u>. Let the person you called hang up first.

<u>Rescue and Transportation</u>. Upon receiving the emergency call, trained professional/paraprofessional personnel are sent to the scene to provide more definitive care. These individuals bring knowledge and the necessary tools to rescue, stabilize, and transport victims.

<u>Hospital Emergency Facilities</u>. At the hospital, further stabilizing care is given and medical procedures are begun by physicians, nurses, and technicians. However, all of the sophisticated equipment and specialized training available at emergency facilities will be of value <u>only</u> if immediate care is given on the scene and the EMS system is activated.

CONTENTS

Unit 1
MOUTH-TO-MOUTH BREATHING

In a respiratory emergency, breathing stops or is so reduced that the body does not get enough oxygen to support life. Causes of respiratory failure include:

- Heart disease.
- Stroke.
- Drowning.
- Airway blocked by food, a foreign object, or the tongue.
- Circulatory collapse caused by shock or bleeding.
- Overdose of drugs.
- Electrocution.
- Toxic gases.
- Suffocation.
- External strangulation, as in hanging.

In this discussion, "mouth-to-mouth breathing" refers also to variations such as mouth-to-nose breathing. Mouth-to-mouth breathing makes air flow in and out of the lungs of a person whose breathing has stopped or has become inadequate. In mouth-to-mouth breathing, you force air from your lungs into the victim's lungs.

Air that you inhale contains about 21% oxygen, and air that you exhale contains about 16% oxygen. In air that you exhale, enough oxygen remains to support life. As long as the other life-supporting body functions are working, mouth-to-mouth breathing will keep a person alive.

Is the Person Conscious?

If someone collapses, find out if he or she is conscious right away. Tap the victim's shoulder firmly or shake the victim gently and shout, "Are you OK?" A person who is conscious will respond and will <u>not</u> have stopped breathing. Check for other problems and keep checking for consciousness. Do not shake the person vigorously if there is any chance of neck or back injury.

If the victim does not respond, shout, "Help!" to get the attention of people who may be able to help you.

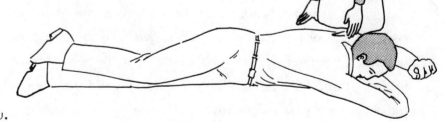

Positioning the Victim

If the victim is unconscious, you will check for breathing and, depending on the victim's condition, you may have to give mouth-to-mouth breathing, correct a blocked airway, or give cardiopulmonary resuscitation (CPR). The victim must be lying on the back for CPR, and mouth-to-mouth breathing is easier to give if the victim is on the back. If the victim is lying face down or in some awkward position, you must consider injuries you can cause or make worse by moving the victim. How did the victim get here? By falling from a high ladder? By being struck by a car? As a result of passing out while having a heart attack or stroke?

If you are fairly sure that the victim collapsed without injuries, you should probably position him or her on the back right away. If you are caring for a victim of a violent accident, however, it is probably better to check for breathing before you move the victim at all. In many cases you can not know for sure what injuries a person has. You must use your best judgment.

Your goal is to roll the victim as a unit, all at once, without twisting any body parts. First, straighten the legs and arms so they won't get in the way. Then roll the victim toward you, onto the back.

This picture shows a method that will work in many cases—support the head and neck with one hand, and pull with the other hand just under the victim's arm. Keep the body from twisting.

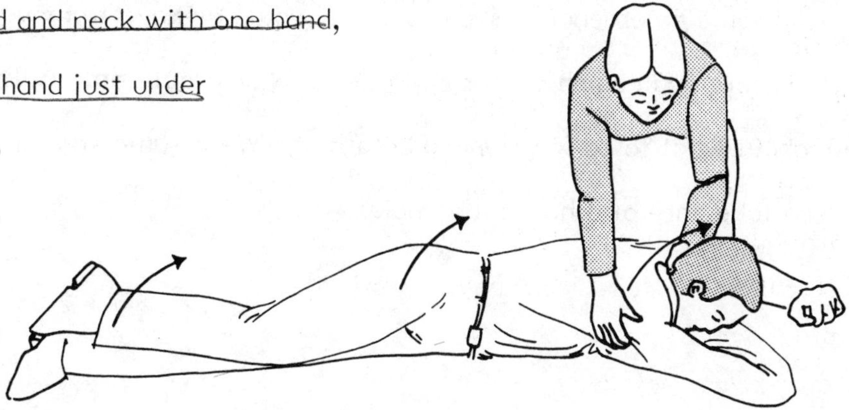

Always check the breathing of an unconscious person right away. You have only a few minutes to save the life of someone whose breathing has stopped. Every moment that you wait makes recovery less likely. Permanent brain damage can occur very quickly, sometimes in less than 4 minutes.

In some emergencies, such as a fire, you may have to move the victim to a safe place before you can check for consciousness or breathing. In this section we are talking only about what to do for stopped breathing. We assume you have learned or will learn how to take care of other emergencies.

The Airway Step

The first step for an unconscious person is the <u>Airway</u> step: <u>tip the head back to open the airway, and check for breathing. Ti</u>p the person's head <u>way back, until the chin points straight up.</u> Tipping the head moves the lower jaw forward, and the tongue is attached to the lower jaw, so tipping the head moves the tongue away from the back of the throat and opens the airway. If <u>you do not tip the head, the tongue may block the airway.</u>

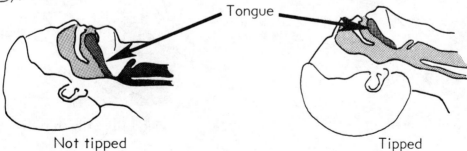

Tongue

Not tipped

Tipped

Place one hand on the victim's forehead and apply firm, backward pressure with the palm. To help tip the head way back, gently lift the victim's neck or chin with your other hand.

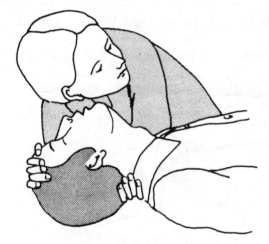

Head tip with neck lift

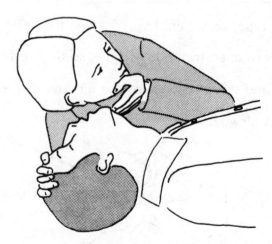

Head tip with chin lift

<u>Head Tip with Neck Lift</u>. There are three important points to remember when you tip the head with the neck lift.

- Apply the major force with the hand that is on the forehead.

- Place the hand under the neck near the base of the skull.

- Support and lift gently with the hand under the neck.

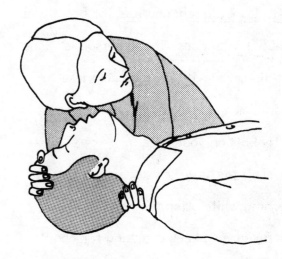

As you tip the head, put your ear down near the mouth and look at the chest. Look, listen, and feel for breathing for about 5 seconds. If the person is breathing, you will see the chest rise and fall, hear air at the mouth and nose, and feel air on your cheek.

This picture shows checking for breathing while using the head tip—neck lift. Be sure to keep checking for about 5 seconds.

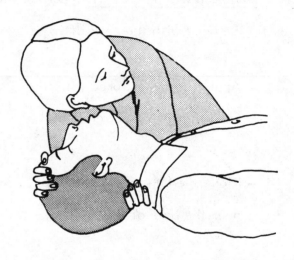

The Airway Step:

Tip Head and Check Breathing

1. What are the two parts of the Airway step?

   _____Tip_____ the head and check for _____breathing_____.

2. Which picture shows how far to tip the head?

   [ ] a.   [x] b.

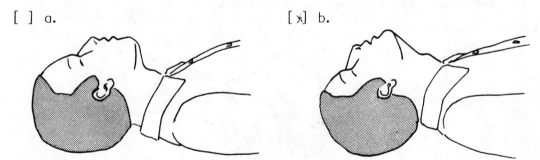

3. When you use the head tip—neck lift, the major force is applied
   with the hand that is

   [x] a. on the forehead.
   [ ] b. under the neck.

Answers:

1. The two parts of the Airway step are <u>tip</u> the head and check for <u>breathing</u>.

2.   b. This picture shows how far to tip the head:

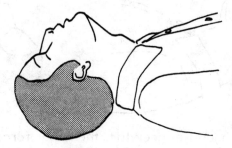

3.   a. The major force is applied with the hand that is on the forehead.

4. Place the hand under the neck near the

[ ] a. shoulders.
[ ] b. base of the skull.

5. Use the hand under the neck to

[ ] a. lift forcefully.
[ ] b. support and lift gently.

6. How do you check for breathing?

[ ] a. Check the pulse at the neck.
[ ] b. Check the pupils of the eyes.
[ ] c. Look at the chest; listen and feel for air coming out of the mouth.

Answers:

4.   b. Place the hand under the neck near the base of the skull.

5.   b. Use the hand under the neck to support and lift gently.

6.   c. Look at the chest; listen and feel for air coming out of the mouth.

<u>Head Tip with Chin Lift</u>. When you tip the head, you can use the neck lift or the chin lift. There are five important points to remember for the chin lift.

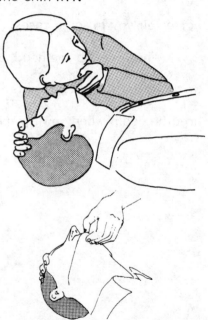

— Apply the major force with the hand on the forehead.

— Place your fingertips under the bony part of the jaw near the chin.

— Support and lift the jaw with your fingertips, but avoid closing the mouth.

— Do not push on the soft tissues of the throat— this may block the airway.

— If necessary, pull the lower lip down slightly with your thumb to keep the mouth open.

How Should You Tip the Head? The head tip–neck lift is well known and has been used successfully for many years. The head tip–chin lift has been shown to produce a better airway in some cases. You should learn both.

When you tip the head, be sure to put your ear near the victim's mouth and look at the chest to check for breathing. Someone who has stopped breathing may start to breathe again when you tip the head.

7.   What is the Airway step? Tip the head and check for breathing for about

[ ]   a. one second.
[ ]   b. 5 seconds.

8.   When you do the head tip—chin lift, place your fingertips under the

[ ]   a. bony part of the jaw near the chin.
[ ]   b. soft part of the throat near the chin.

9.   Which picture shows how to do the chin lift?

[ ] a.   [ ] b. 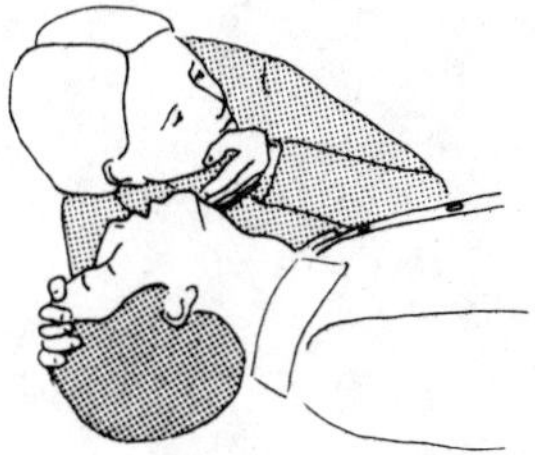   [ ] c.

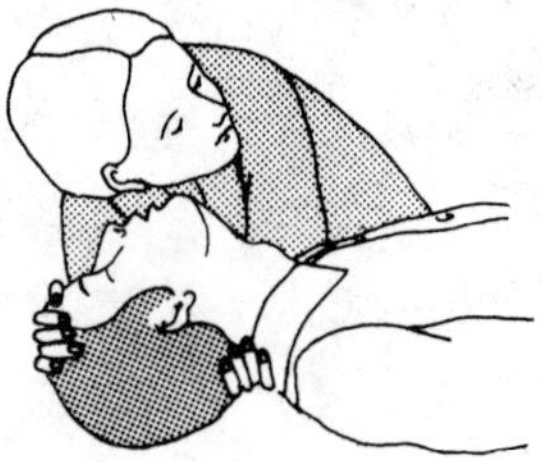

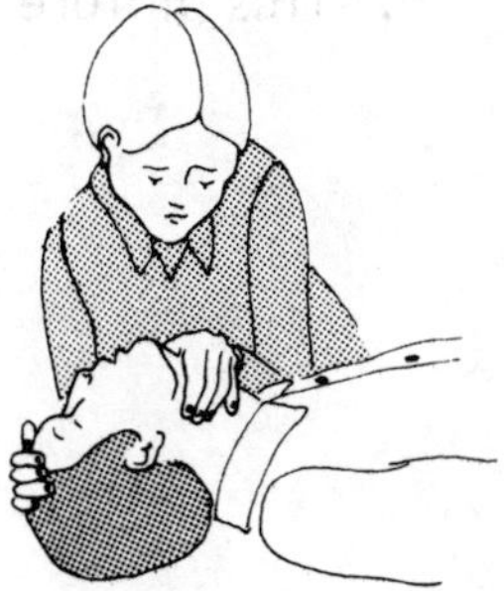

Answers:

7. b. The Airway step is to tip the head and check for breathing for about 5 seconds.

8. a. When you do the head tip—chin lift, place your fingertips under the bony part of the jaw near the chin.

9. b. This picture shows how to do the chin lift.

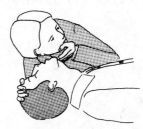

The Quick Step

If the person is not breathing, give 4 quick, full breaths. This is called the Quick step.

Keep the head tipped. Pinch the nose so air will not come out the nose when you blow into the mouth. Take a deep breath and open your mouth wide. Cover the victim's mouth with your mouth. Make a good seal.

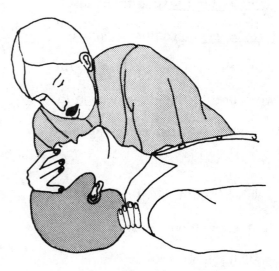

<u>Give 4 big breaths as fast as you can, without letting the lungs deflate between breaths.</u> Remove your mouth from the victim's mouth between breaths just long enough to get a fast gulp of air for the next breath.

Give breaths right on top of each other, without pauses. This expands the lungs fully and gives a lot of oxygen quickly.

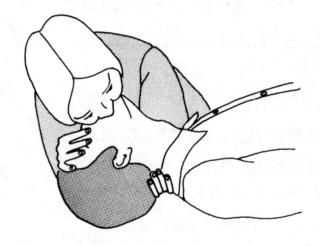

The Quick Step:

4 Quick Breaths

10. Fill in the two parts of the Airway step:

    Airway: _____ and _____

11. The 4 quick breaths should be

    [ ] a. small breaths.
    [ ] b. full breaths.

12. How long do you pause between each of the 4 quick breaths?

    [ ] a. About 3 seconds between each breath.
    [ ] b. Only long enough to get a breath.

Answers:

10. Airway: <u>tip the head</u> and <u>check for breathing</u>.

11. b. Give <u>full</u> breaths.

12. b. Pause <u>only long enough to get a breath</u> between each of the 4 quick breaths.

The Check Step

After you give 4 quick breaths, check the pulse and check for breathing again. This is called the <u>Check</u> step. To help remember the first steps for an unconscious person, use the phrase "A Quick Check".

<u>A</u> = <u>A</u>irway: Tip the head and check for breathing.

<u>Quick</u> = Give 4 <u>quick</u>, full breaths.

<u>Check</u> = <u>Check</u> the pulse and breathing.

Check the pulse on the side of the neck near you. Keep the head tipped with your hand on the forehead. Place the fingertips of your other hand on the Adam's apple, then slide your fingers into the groove at the side of the neck. _Check the pulse and breathing for at least 5 seconds but no more than 10 seconds._

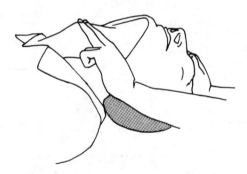

Start here.

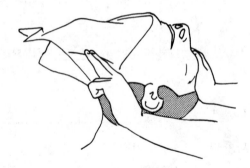

Check pulse here.

Find your own neck pulse now.

13. Where do you find the pulse?

[ ] a. In the groove at the side of the neck.
[ ] b. On top of the Adam's apple.

14. Check the pulse and breathing for at least _____ seconds.

15. What are the steps for A Quick Check?

A = Airway: _____ and check _____.

Quick = Give _____.

Check = Check the _____ and check _____.

Answers:

13.   a. Find the pulse in the groove at the <u>side</u> of the neck.

14.   Check the pulse and breathing for at least <u>5</u> seconds.

15.   The steps for A Quick Check are:

A = Airway: <u>Tip the head</u> and <u>check for breathing</u>.

Quick = Give <u>4 quick breaths</u>.

Check = Check the <u>pulse</u> and <u>breathing</u>.

Please read about the EMS system on the inside front cover of this book now, if you have not done so already. Then continue on this page.

If the person is not breathing but <u>has a pulse, give mouth-to-mouth breathing.</u> If the person is not breathing and <u>does not have</u> a pulse, cardiopulmonary resuscitation (CPR) is needed and the <u>EMS system should be activated.</u> If you have not been trained in CPR, give mouth-to-mouth breathing. The heart may be beating even though you did not find a pulse, so mouth-to-mouth breathing may keep the person alive. If you are not scheduled to study CPR, sign up to do so soon.

Get ready to give more breaths this way:

1) Be sure the head is still tipped.
2) Pinch the nose shut again.
3) Take a deep breath, open your mouth wide, and make a tight seal over the victim's mouth.

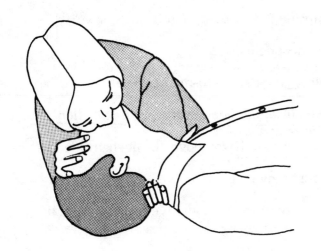 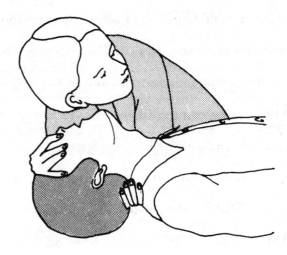

Blow to fill up the lungs.   Listen and feel for air.
Watch the chest rise.   Watch the chest fall.

Do these steps once every 5 seconds. It may help to count, "One, one-thousand;

two, one-thousand; three, one-thousand; four, one-thousand; b-r-e-a-t-h-e."

16. How do you count for one breath every 5 seconds?

[ ] a. "One-and, two-and, three-and, four-and, b-r-e-a-t-h-e."
[ ] b. "One, one-thousand; two, one-thousand; three, one-thousand; four, one-thousand; b-r-e-a-t-h-e."

✓ 17. When you take a breath, turn your head to look at the victim's

[ ] a. chest.
[ ] b. forehead.

18. What phrase will help you to remember the first steps for an unconscious person?

✓

_____   _____   _____

Answers:

16. b. Count, "One, one-thousand; two, one-thousand; three, one-thousand; four, one-thousand; b-r-e-a-t-h-e," for one breath every 5 seconds.

√ 17. a. Turn your head to look at the victim's <u>chest</u> while you take another breath.

√ 18. Give an unconscious person <u>A Quick Check</u>.

PRACTICE SESSION 1

Now you are ready to practice mouth-to-mouth breathing. Please take the following steps. Check each one when you complete it.

____ 1. Read pages 1-32 through 1-39 to see what you will be practicing.

____ 2. Sign up for Practice Session 1.

If you cannot practice right away, continue reading at page 1-40 after you have done the above steps.

Directions for Practice With a Manikin

Have a practice partner read the checklist to you when you practice at first.
Then have your partner watch you practice without reading aloud. Your partner should
help you to improve your performance and check your checklist in the "Partner check"
boxes when you can do the steps correctly. If you have questions, review the workbook.
If you need more help, ask your instructor.

Some practice manikins are more difficult to work with than humans. Do not
be discouraged if you find it hard to tip the head, pinch the nose, or make a good seal
on the mouth. If you have trouble making a good seal, do _not_ push hard with your mouth.
Pushing hard does not work better, and you will bruise your mouth.

If a manikin is available but a partner is not, please begin to practice alone. When
a partner becomes available, work together.

Directions for Practice Without a Manikin

If you do not have a manikin in your class, practice with two other students. One student is the rescuer, the second is the victim, and the third reads the directions and checks the rescuer's checklist. Rotate so that each student plays each role.

When using a class member as a victim, DO NOT MAKE MOUTH-TO-MOUTH CONTACT. Go through all the motions, but place your mouth near the victim's cheek when you blow.

Mouth-to-Mouth Breathing
Using the Head Tip—Neck Lift

Partner Check [ ]   Instructor Check [ ]

For practice, find another student's pulse at the neck.

Check consciousness.
– Rescuer taps shoulder and shouts, "Are you OK?"
– Rescuer says, "Unconscious," and shouts, "Help!"

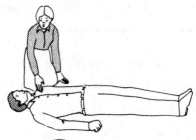

[ ] [ ]   Airway step: tip head and check breathing for about 5 seconds. Use head tip—neck lift.
– One hand on forehead.
– Other hand under neck, near base of skull.
– Head tipped <u>way</u> back.
– Look at chest, ear <u>near</u> victim's mouth.
– Rescuer says, "Not breathing."

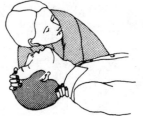

Go on to the next page without stopping.

[ ]   [ ]   Quick step: 4 quick breaths.
                – Nose pinched, head tipped.
                – Open mouth wide and make a tight seal.
                – Remove mouth from victim's mouth to
                   get breaths.
                – No pause between breaths.
                – Give _big_ breaths quickly.

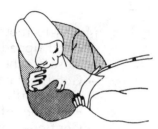

[ ]   [ ]   Check step: check pulse and breathing.
                – Head tipped, look at chest, ear _near_
                   victim's mouth.
                – Check pulse on side of neck near rescuer.
                – Check pulse and breathing for at least 5
                   but not more than 10 seconds.
                – Rescuer says, "Has pulse, still not breathing.
                   Someone call 911 or 0 for help!"

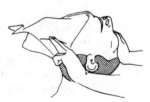

Go on to the next page without stopping.

Mouth-to-mouth breathing.
- Head tipped.
- Nose pinched.
- Good seal on mouth.
- One breath every 5 seconds.
- Full lung inflations.
- Continue until partner or instructor says to stop (about 12 breaths).

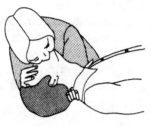

[ ] [ ] DECISION MAKING. After you have mastered the above steps, practice what you would do if the victim is breathing at the Airway step or at the Check step. To do this, have your partner tell you what you find when you check for breathing. Your partner should tell you "Breathing," or "Not breathing," when you are checking, not beforehand. Be prepared to have your instructor do the same during your checkout.

If you wish to check your overall speed, time these three pages from the beginning. The total time should be 80—120 seconds when the victim is not breathing. When the rescuer can do these steps correctly, go on to the next page and have the same rescuer practice mouth-to-mouth breathing with the head tip—chin lift.

Mouth-to-Mouth Breathing

Using the Head Tip–Chin Lift

Partner Check [ ] Instructor Check [ ]

Check consciousness.
- Rescuer taps shoulder and shouts, "Are you OK?"
- Rescuer says, "Unconscious," and shouts, "Help!"

[ ] [ ] Airway step: tip head and check breathing for about 5 seconds. Use head tip–chin lift.
- One hand on forehead.
- Fingertips of other hand under bony part of jaw near chin.
- Lift jaw, avoid closing mouth.
- Head tipped <u>way</u> back.
- Look at chest, ear <u>near</u> victim's mouth.
- Rescuer says, "Not breathing."

Go on to the next page without stopping.

[ ] [ ] Quick step: 4 quick breaths.
— Nose pinched, head tipped.
— Open mouth wide and make a tight seal.
— Remove mouth from victim's mouth to
   get breaths.
— No pause between breaths.
— Give <u>big</u> breaths quickly.

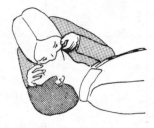

[ ] [ ] Check step: check pulse and breathing.
— Head tipped, look at chest, ear <u>near</u>
   victim's mouth.
— Check pulse on side of neck near rescuer.
— <u>Check pulse and breathing for at least 5</u>
   <u>but not more than 10 seconds.</u>
— Rescuer says, "Has pulse, still not breathing.
   Someone call 911 or 0 for help!"

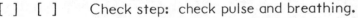

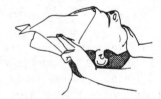

Go on to the next page without stopping.

[ ] [ ]   Mouth-to-mouth breathing.
                — Head tipped.
                — Nose pinched.
                — Good seal on mouth.
                — One breath every 5 seconds.
                — Full lung inflations.
                — Continue until partner or instructor
                   says to stop (about 12 breaths).

[ ] [ ]   DECISION MAKING. Repeat the above steps and have your partner tell
                you "Breathing," or "Not breathing," when you check for breathing. Be
                prepared to have your instructor do the same during your checkout.

    If you wish to check your overall speed, time these three pages from the beginning.
The total time should be 80—120 seconds when the victim is not breathing. When the
rescuer can do these steps correctly, clean the manikin and change places so another
partner can practice, starting on page 1—34. When all partners are ready, ask the
instructor for a checkout.

Final Instructor Checkout: _____

Mouth-to-Nose Breathing

Sometimes you cannot make a good seal over the mouth:

- Air may leak out when you blow.

- The victim's mouth or jaw may be injured.

- The victim's jaws may be shut tight so that you cannot open the mouth to give a breath.

- Your mouth may be too small.

If you cannot make a good mouth-to-mouth seal, give mouth-to-nose breathing.

Hand positions for mouth-to-nose breathing:

Step 1: Tip the head. Use either the
               neck lift or the chin lift.

Step 2: Close the mouth.

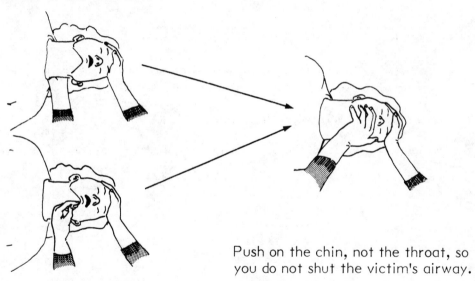

Push on the chin, not the throat, so
you do not shut the victim's airway.

Blow into the nose.

Then open the mouth and listen for air. Watch the chest fall.

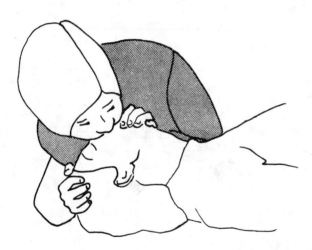

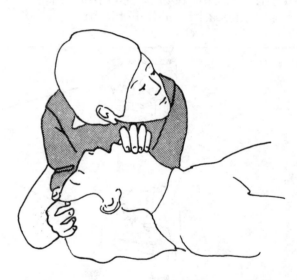

19. While you blow into the <u>nose</u>, what do you do with the person's mouth?

[ ] a. Close the mouth.
[ ] b. Open the mouth.

20. Fill in the first steps for mouth-to-mouth (or mouth-to-nose) breathing:

A = Airway: _____ and _____.

Quick = _____.

Check = _____ and _____.

Answers:

19.   a. <u>Close</u> the person's mouth while you blow into the nose.

20.   A = Airway: <u>Tip the head and check breathing</u>.

Quick = <u>Give 4 quick breaths</u>.

Check = <u>Check the pulse and breathing</u>.

Air in the Stomach

When you are giving mouth-to-mouth breathing, the victim's stomach may fill up with air. Air in the stomach can push against the lungs, making it difficult or impossible to give full breaths. You can expel the air by pushing on the stomach, but this is dangerous to do because the victim may vomit and inhale the vomit into the lungs. When you give breaths, try to blow just hard enough to make the chest rise, because you are likely to force air into the stomach if you blow too hard.

If the stomach is bulging with air and you can not inflate the lungs, take these steps:

1) Turn the victim on one side.
2) Push on the stomach with your hand between the rib cage and the waist.
3) Clean out the mouth if the victim vomits.
4) Roll the victim onto the back and continue mouth-to-mouth breathing.

Take these steps only if air in the stomach is keeping you from giving breaths.

Dentures

It may be hard to make a good mouth-to-mouth seal on a person who wears dentures (false teeth) if the dentures slip out of place and allow the lips to cave in. Try to hold dentures in place by holding the chin up with the chin lift.

If you can not hold the dentures in place, take them out and give mouth-to-mouth breathing or mouth-to-nose breathing.

21.   If a victim seems to have air in the stomach, but you <u>can</u> give full breaths, should you try to remove the air?

[ ]   a. No, it is dangerous to push on the stomach. Try to remove the air only if you can not give full breaths.
[ ]   b. Yes, always remove air when the stomach bulges.

22.   Which method of tipping the head may help you hold a victim's dentures in place?

[ ]   a. Head tip—neck lift.
[ ]   b. Head tip—chin lift.

Answers:

21. a. No, it is dangerous to push on the stomach. Try to remove the
         air only if you can not give full breaths.

22. b. The head tip—chin lift may help you hold a victim's dentures in
         place.

Mouth-to-Stoma Breathing

About 25,000 persons in the United States have had part or all of the larynx (voice box) removed by surgery. These people breathe through an opening in the front of the neck (a stoma), so mouth-to-stoma breathing is used for them.

A person with a stoma may have a passage from the lungs to the mouth and nose, so you may need to block the mouth and nose when you blow in the stoma. If the lungs do not inflate when you blow in the stoma, block the mouth and nose with your hand.

A person may wear a breathing tube in a stoma. If the tube is clogged, it is safe to remove it with the fingers to open the airway. Send the tube with the victim to the hospital, or allow the victim to clean and replace it. The rescuer should not replace the tube.

When giving mouth-to-stoma breathing,

- do not tip the head. Keep the head and neck straight.

- check breathing with your ear near the stoma.

- give breaths with your mouth sealed over the stoma.

- block the mouth and nose if air escapes from them when you blow in the stoma.

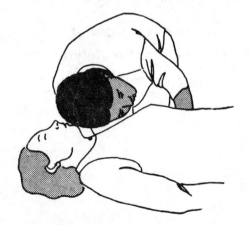 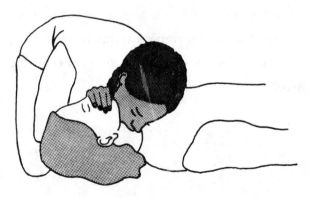

23. How do you place the head for mouth-to-stoma breathing?

[ ] a. Tipped back.
[ ] b. Straight.

24. Where is a stoma located?

[ ] a. The front of the neck.
[ ] b. The side of the neck.
[ ] c. The back of the neck.

Answers:

23.   b.   Keep the head <u>straight</u> for mouth-to-stoma breathing.

24.   a.   A stoma is at the <u>front</u> of the neck.

Types of Airway Obstruction

<u>Anatomic</u> <u>obstruction</u> is caused by the tongue dropping back and blocking the throat, or by tissues in the throat swelling and interfering with breathing. Narrowing of the airway may be caused by disease, burns, and injury.

Tipping the head will usually open the airway. If you cannot inflate the lungs when you try to give breaths, <u>retip the head</u> and try again. You may not have tipped the head far enough at first.

<u>Mechanical</u> <u>obstruction</u> is blockage of the airway by an object or by fluids such as mucus, blood, saliva, or vomit collecting in the back of the throat. Food is the most common mechanical obstruction in adults.

There are a number of causes of choking on food. Consumption of too much alcohol deadens sensations in the mouth; false teeth reduce normal sensations in the mouth; large bites of poorly chewed food are hard to swallow. Surprisingly large pieces of unchewed food are found blocking the throats of people who have choked to death.

The tongue and fluids such as blood or vomit are likely to block the airway of an unconscious person who is lying flat on the back. Most people who need mouth-to-mouth breathing do not have a foreign object blocking the airway. If you cannot get air to go into the lungs, retip the head and try again to give breaths. If that still does not work, an object may be blocking the airway. Units 4 and 5 describe how to remove an object from the airway.

25. In which position is the tongue more likely to block the airway of an unconscious person?

[ ] a. Lying on the side.
[ ] b. Lying on the back.

26. If you cannot get air to go into the lungs,

[ ] a. retip the head and try again to give breaths.
[ ] b. do the check step.

Answers:

25.   b. The tongue is more likely to block the airway if the person is <u>lying on the back</u>.

26.   a. <u>Retip the head</u> and try again to give breaths if you cannot get air to go into the lungs.

Jutting the Jaw

If a person was in an accident that might have caused a broken neck or back, or if bones in the face may be broken, do not tip the head. You may be able to give breaths after pushing the jaw forward (jutting or thrusting the jaw) without tipping the head.

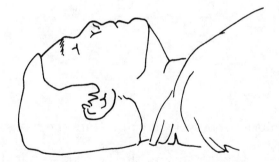

Jaw in normal position

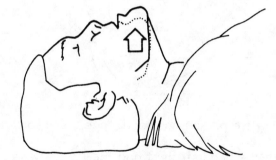

Jaw pushed forward

Place your fingers on the corners of the jaw and push the jaw forward. Keep the jaw forward as you give breaths. Let your cheek puff out to block the nose when you blow.

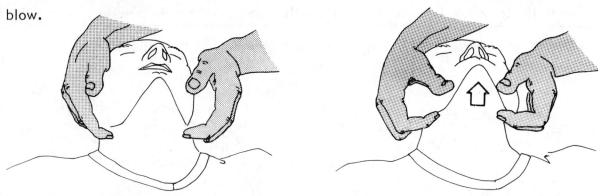

If a person has head, face, neck, or back injuries, and you cannot inflate the lungs with the head straight and the jaw forward, it may be necessary to tip the head as a last resort. To do this, tip it only slightly—just enough to allow you to inflate the lungs.

Followup Care

After a victim starts to breathe again, watch to be sure he or she keeps breathing.

Give care to prevent shock:

- Keep the victim lying down and at a comfortable temperature.

- Raise the feet and legs if moving the legs does not cause injury or pain.

- Raise the head and shoulders if the victim has trouble breathing or has a head injury. Do not put the head on a pillow, because this may bend the neck and block the airway.

- Call a doctor or ambulance, or take the victim to a hospital or life support unit.

In some cases, a person can be kept alive by mouth-to-mouth breathing but will not start breathing without medical treatment. Mouth-to-mouth breathing may be needed for a very long time. Keep giving mouth-to-mouth breathing until the victim recovers, someone else who can give mouth-to-mouth breathing effectively takes over, a physician assumes responsibility, medical personnel take over, or you become too exhausted to continue.

Unit 2
ONE-RESCUER CPR

The heart and lungs work together. The air that is breathed into the lungs gives oxygen to the blood. The heart circulates blood, carrying oxygen to the brain and to the rest of the body. If a person stops breathing, the heart may keep beating for a short time. In this case, mouth-to-mouth breathing is needed. If a heart attack, illness, or injury makes the heart stop beating (cardiac arrest), breathing will not continue. In this case, cardiopulmonary resuscitation is needed.

In cardiopulmonary resuscitation, cardio refers to the heart and pulmonary refers to the lungs. CPR is the combination of mouth-to-mouth breathing, which supplies oxygen to the lungs, and chest compressions, which circulate blood. By giving CPR, you breathe and circulate blood for a person whose heart and lungs have stopped working.

The most common signals that someone is having a heart attack are feelings of uncomfortable pressure, squeezing, fullness, or pain in the center of the chest. Sometimes the pain is in the upper abdomen and seems to be indigestion. Pain may travel out from the center of the chest to the shoulders, arms, neck, and jaw. Other signals are sweating, nausea, shortness of breath, and a feeling of weakness.

Anyone who has persistent signals of heart attack should get medical care at once. Call the paramedics or rescue squad or take the person to a hospital right away. If you think you may be going to have a heart attack, get help immediately. Have someone take you to a hospital if possible.

There are a number of factors that either are known to increase the risk of heart attack or are strongly suspected of contributing to the risk of heart attack. Here are some ways you can reduce the risk of heart attack:

- Blood pressure. If your blood pressure is above normal, get medical help in reducing it.

- Weight. Avoid becoming overweight. If you are overweight, reduce!

- Smoking. Don't. Smoking is a major contributor to heart and artery disease as well as to lung cancer.

- Exercise. Get regular exercise that involves your heart and lungs, such as walking, swimming, cycling, or jogging. Don't start to do vigorous exercise without gradually working up to it.

- Diet. Reduce saturated fats and cholesterol, increase polyunsaturated fats. Avoid large amounts of salt and sugar.

- Medical checkups. Get regular checkups to identify possible risk factors such as high blood pressure and diabetes.

Many of these factors work together, such as weight, exercise, and diet. To make safe and effective large changes in most risk factors, you should have medical advice.

Chest Compressions

CPR is the combination of mouth-to-mouth breathing and chest compressions.
Chest compressions circulate blood by pressing the heart between the sternum
(breastbone) and the backbone.

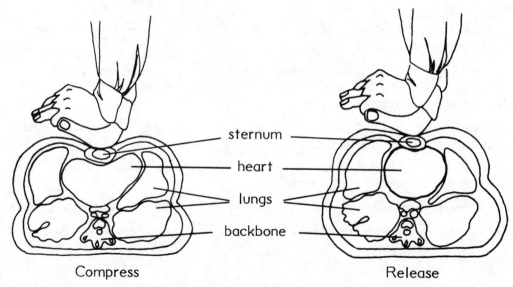

| |
| sternum |
| heart |
| lungs |
| backbone |

Compress   Release

The sternum (breastbone) runs down the front of the chest. The ribs join the sternum in front. The xiphoid (ZI-foyd) is the lower tip of the sternum.

When you give chest compressions, you push on the lower half of the sternum, above the xiphoid. Never push directly on the xiphoid, because you may injure the victim.

Find your own xiphoid now.

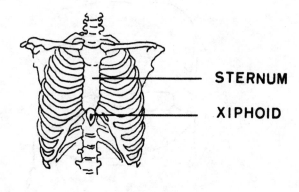

STERNUM

XIPHOID

<u>Finding Where to Give Chest Compressions</u>. Find the lower edge of the victim's rib cage on the side nearer you. Use your hand that is nearer the victim's feet.

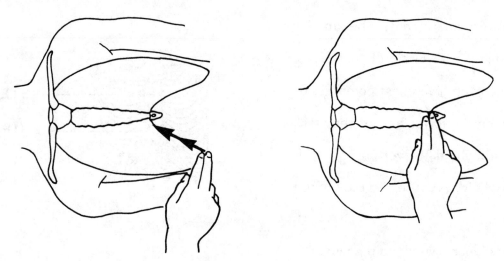

With the middle and index fingers, trace the edge of the ribs up to the notch where the ribs meet the sternum. This is in the center of the lower chest.

Keep your middle finger on the notch and place your index finger next to it on the lower end of the sternum. Put the heel of your other hand on the sternum next to your fingers. If you push on the xiphoid by mistake, it may bend in and injure the liver. It is better to be too high on the sternum than too low.

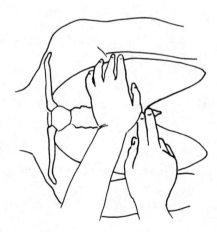

Put your other hand on top. Keep your fingers off the chest. You are more likely to break ribs if you push with your fingers. You may

lace your fingers . . . hold them up . . . or grasp your wrist with your other hand.

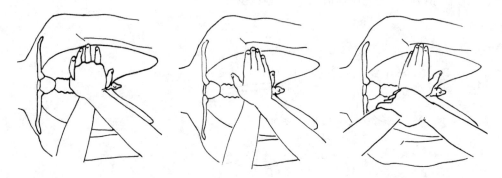

Most people can keep their fingers off the chest if they lace them together, but some find that lacing them does not work. Use the method that works best for you.

1. The first step in finding where to give compressions is to

[ ] a. trace the lower edge of the rib cage to the notch where the ribs meet the sternum.
[ ] b. find the top of the sternum.

2. The second step is to measure up

[ ] a. 3 finger-widths from the middle finger on the notch.
[ ] b. one finger-width from the middle finger on the notch.

3. What do you do with your fingers when you push?

[ ] a. Push with your fingers, too.
[ ] b. Hold your fingers off the victim's chest.

Answers:

1.   a. Trace the lower edge of the rib cage to the notch where the ribs meet the sternum.

2.   b. The second step is to measure up one finger-width from the middle finger on the notch.

3.   b. Hold your fingers <u>off the victim's chest</u> when you push.

"Stand" on your knees, don't sit on your heels. Place your knees about shoulder-width apart. With your shoulders directly over the sternum and your hands along the middle line of your body, push straight down. Use your body weight. Keep your elbows straight.

When you push, bend from your hips, not your knees. This makes it easier to push straight down. If you rock back and forth on your knees, you will not push straight.

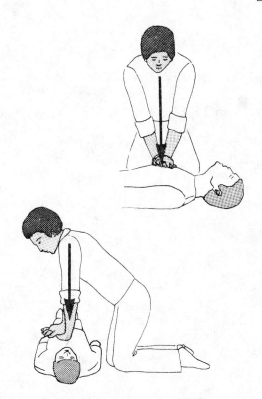

Push straight down, with your fingers pointing across the victim's chest away from you. If you put your hands at an angle, you will push more on the ends of the ribs where they join the sternum. This can injure the victim.

Compress the chest of an adult at least 4 centimeters (1 1/2 to 2 inches). Push very smoothly. Do not jerk. Do not stop at the top or at the bottom. Keep your hands resting lightly on the victim's chest between compressions.

Compress the chest at a rate of 80 compressions per minute when giving one-rescuer CPR to an adult. To help you give compressions at the rate of 80 per minute, count aloud, "One-and, two-and, three-and," and so forth, while you are learning.

4. How do you push on a victim's chest?

[ ] a. Straight down.
[ ] b. At an angle.

5. How far do you compress the chest of an adult?

[ ] a. At least 4 centimeters (1 1/2 to 2 inches).
[ ] b. At least one centimeter (1/4 to 1/2 inch).

6. At what rate do you give chest compressions to an adult in one-rescuer CPR?

[ ] a. 60 per minute.
[ ] b. 80 per minute.
[ ] c. 100 per minute.

Answers:

4.   a. Push <u>straight down</u> on the victim's chest.

5.   a. Compress the chest of an adult at least <u>4 centimeters</u> (1 1/2 to 2 inches).

6.   b. Give chest compressions to an adult at a rate of <u>80 per minute</u> in one-rescuer CPR.

7.   How do you give chest compressions?

[ ]   a. Smoothly and regularly.
[ ]   b. With a quick jerk.

8.   Where do you put your hands when you finish each chest compression?

[ ]   a. 2 to 3 inches above the victim's chest.
[ ]   b. Resting lightly on the victim's chest.

9.   When compressing the chest, keep your elbows

[ ]   a. straight.
[ ]   b. bent slightly.

10.   How do you count for a rate of 80 compressions per minute?

[ ]   a. "One, one-thousand; two, one-thousand; . . ."
[ ]   b. "One-and, two-and, three-and, . . ."

Answers:

7.   a. Give chest compressions <u>smoothly and regularly</u>.

8.   b. Your hands should <u>rest lightly</u> on the victim's chest.

9.   a. Keep your elbows <u>straight</u> when compressing the chest.

10.   b. For a rate of 80, count, "One-and, two-and, three-and, . . ."

When you give CPR, the victim's head should be at the level of the heart or slightly lower than the heart. If the head is higher than the heart, blood will not flow up to the brain.

The victim must be on a firm surface. If the victim is on a soft bed or in the water, chest compressions will not press the heart between the backbone and the sternum. Get the victim onto a firm surface, such as the ground or the floor. If the victim is in a bed and hard to move, put something firm, such as a board, under the victim.

As soon as possible, elevate (raise) the feet and legs of a victim who is being given CPR. This helps blood return to the heart. Do not stop giving CPR to elevate the legs—have another person do it.

Combining Chest Compressions and Mouth-to-Mouth Breathing

In one-rescuer CPR, give 15 compressions at a rate of 80 per minute. Then give 2 quick, full breaths without a pause—the same way you give breaths in the Quick step.

Keep repeating 15 compressions, 2 breaths; 15 compressions, 2 breaths . . . Each time you begin 15 compressions, measure up quickly from the notch.

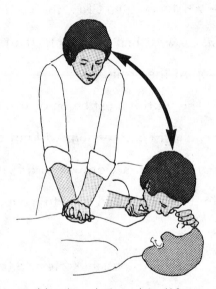

Use head tip—chin lift or head tip—neck lift.

11. In one-rescuer CPR, what is the pattern of compressions and breaths?

[ ] a. 5 compressions, then 1 breath.
[ ] b. 15 compressions, then 2 breaths.

12. In one-rescuer CPR, should there be a pause between the 2 quick, full breaths?

[ ] a. Yes.
[ ] b. No.

13. What kind of surface should the victim be on when receiving CPR?

[ ] a. Hard.
[ ] b. Soft.

14. Which positions of the victim are acceptable for CPR?

[ ] a. Body level or head higher than the heart.
[ ] b. Body level or head lower than the heart.

Answers:

11.　b.　In one-rescuer CPR, you give 15 compressions, then 2 breaths.

12.　b.　<u>No</u>, do not pause between the 2 quick, full breaths.

13.　a.　The surface should be <u>hard</u>.

14.　b.　The victim may be <u>level</u> or have the head <u>lower than</u> the heart.

15. Which picture shows how to give chest compressions?

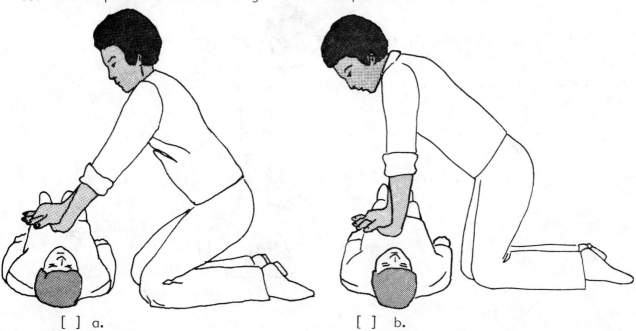

[ ] a.

[ ] b.

Answer:

15. b. Give chest compressions this way:

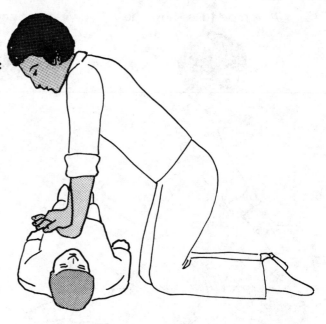

PRACTICE SESSION 2

Please take the following steps. Check each one when you complete it.

____ 1. Read pages 2–24 through 2–29 to see what you will be practicing.

____ 2. Sign up for Practice Session 2.

IMPORTANT: <u>Never</u> practice CPR on anyone. If you give CPR correctly, you are less likely to injure a victim. However, CPR can break ribs and cause other damage, even when given correctly.

This session requires a manikin and one partner. When you practice, have your partner read the checklist aloud and check your performance. Start to practice chest compressions by yourself if a manikin is available but a partner is not. If you cannot practice right away, continue reading at page 2–30 until you can practice.

Preparatory Practice

First you will practice chest compressions without mouth-to-mouth breathing. Then you will practice one-rescuer CPR. Remember that CPR always requires both chest compressions and mouth-to-mouth breathing.

[ ] Find hand position for compressions.
- Kneel beside victim, knees a shoulder-width apart.
- Find lower edge of ribs with hand nearer victim's feet.
- Trace up to notch. (1)
- Measure up one finger width from the middle finger. (2)
- Heel of hand beside fingers. (3)
- Other hand on top. (4) Lacing of fingers is optional.

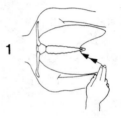
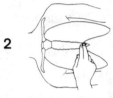
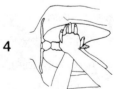
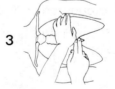

Check position of arms and body.

— Elbows straight. Partner
  checks by looking across
  manikin's chest at rescuer.

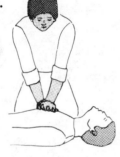

— Shoulders over sternum, arms straight
  up and down. Partner checks by looking
  from head or feet of manikin.

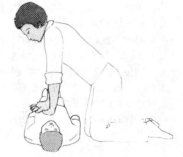

Take turns until all partners can find the hand position and body position quickly.

Partner
Check

[ ]   Give chest compressions.
— Measure up from notch for each
   group of 15 compressions.
— Chest compressed 4 cm
   (1 1/2 to 2 inches).
— Rate of 80 compressions per minute.
   Practice slowly at first.
— Count aloud, "One-and, two-and, . . ."
— Smooth compressions.
— Fingertips not touching chest.
— Bend at hips, not knees.
— Hands rest lightly on chest
   between compressions.
— Elbows straight.
— Shoulders over sternum.

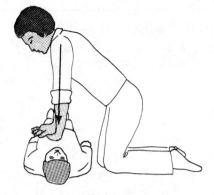

   Take turns practicing until you can give several groups of 15 compressions in 10 to
12 seconds without needing correction from your partner.

One-Rescuer CPR

[ ] [ ]   Check consciousness.
— Rescuer taps shoulder and shouts, "Are you OK?"
— Rescuer says, "Unconscious," and shouts, "Help!"

[ ] [ ]   Airway step: tip head and check breathing for about 5 seconds.
— Head tipped, look at chest, ear near victim's mouth.
— Rescuer says, "Not breathing."

[ ] [ ]   Quick step: 4 quick breaths.
— Nose pinched, head tipped.
— Remove mouth from victim's mouth to get breaths.
— No pause between big breaths.

[ ] [ ]   Check step: check pulse and breathing.
— Head tipped, look at chest, ear near victim's mouth.
— Check pulse on side of neck near rescuer.
— Check pulse and breathing for at least 5 but not more than 10 seconds.
— Rescuer says, "No breathing, no pulse. Someone call 911 or 0 for help!"

Go on to the next page without stopping.

Partner Check [ ] Instructor Check [ ] One-rescuer CPR. Four cycles of 15 compressions and 2 breaths.
- Measure up from notch for each group of 15 compressions.
- Correct hand position, elbows straight, shoulders over sternum.
- Count aloud, "One-and, two-and, . . ."
- Smoothly compress and release at rate of 80, no bouncing.
- Lean down for breaths instead of sliding toward head on your knees.
- Tip head and give 2 full breaths in 4 seconds.

[ ] [ ] Check pulse and breathing for 5 seconds.
- Head tipped.
- Ear near mouth.

[ ] [ ] Continue one-rescuer CPR.
One cycle; start with two breaths.

Partner Check [ ]   Instructor Check [ ]

DECISION MAKING. After you have mastered the steps on pages 2–27 and 2–28, practice what you would do for a victim who is breathing or has a pulse at one of the checks. Have your partner tell you what you find, following the plans below, but in mixed order so you will not know what to expect.

— Plan A. At Airway step, partner says, "The victim is breathing." Rescuer keeps head tipped, does not give mouth-to-mouth breathing, checks again soon.
— Plan B. At Airway step, partner says, "Not breathing." At Check step, partner says, "Not breathing, does have a pulse." Rescuer gives mouth-to-mouth breathing.
— Plan C. At Airway step, partner says "Not breathing." At Check step, partner says, "Not breathing, no pulse." Rescuer gives one-rescuer CPR.

The steps, following Plan C, should take 90–135 seconds. Clean the manikin when you change places. When both partners can do these steps correctly, ask the instructor for a checkout.

Final Instructor Checkout: _LQU_____

Checking the Pulse

The first time you check an unconscious person's pulse is during the Check step, just after giving 4 quick breaths. Check for at least 5 but no more than 10 seconds.

- If you find a pulse and breathing, keep checking the pulse and breathing.

- If you find a pulse but no breathing, give mouth-to-mouth breathing. Activate the EMS system. Check the pulse frequently.

- If you find no pulse, start CPR. Activate the EMS system.

You must start CPR immediately, but you must also get help through the EMS system. If someone else is present, he or she should be sent for help. In an area where there are telephones, it is usually effective to dial 911 or 0 (operator) for help. In an area without telephones, you will have to use your best judgment.

If you are alone, call aloud for help and then give CPR for one minute. Then, if no help has come and you are near other people or a telephone, quickly seek help. You must balance the risk of pausing in CPR against the risk of never getting help while giving CPR. The purpose of CPR is to keep the victim alive until medical help is obtained or until the heart and lungs start working again. In most cases when CPR is needed, the victim must be transferred directly to medical care while CPR is being given, in order to survive.

Once you have started CPR, check the pulse and breathing after the first minute and every few minutes after that. Check right after you give breaths. Do not stop CPR for more than 5 seconds to check the pulse and breathing. Also check the pulse if you see signs of recovery, such as small movements, return of reflexes such as swallowing, and improved skin color in persons who have light skin.

- If you find no pulse, continue CPR. When you start one-rescuer CPR again after checking the pulse, give two breaths first, then compressions.

- If you find a pulse but no breathing, give mouth-to-mouth breathing. Check the pulse and breathing frequently.

- If you find a pulse and breathing, keep checking the pulse and breathing. Get the person to a hospital or life-support unit quickly.

16. After you have given CPR for about a minute, stop to check the pulse and breathing. After that, check once every

[ ] a. 5 or 10 minutes.
[ ] b. few minutes.

17. When you start one-rescuer CPR again after stopping to check the pulse, start with

[ ] a. 2 breaths.
[ ] b. 15 compressions.

Answers:

16.   b. Check the pulse and breathing every few minutes after the first check.

17.   a. After checking the pulse, start one-rescuer CPR again with 2 breaths.

Unit 3
REVIEW

This unit will help you review for your final test. Answer the questions, then check your answers. The answers begin on page 3—5. If you can't remember an answer or are not sure of it, check back in the workbook before you answer.

Unit I

1. What is the phrase you learned to help you remember the first steps for an

    unconscious person? _____

2. What are the three steps that the phrase names?

    _____

    _____

    _____

3. How many breaths do you give at first? _____

4. What kind of breaths are they? _____

5.   After you give the first breaths, what do you do? _____

6.   What is the rate of breaths in mouth-to-mouth breathing for an adult?

_____

7.   When might you use mouth-to-nose breathing? _____

_____

8.   When would you try to give breaths without tipping the head? _____

_____

Unit 2

9. What is the rate of compressions in one-rescuer CPR? _____

10. What is the pattern of breaths and compressions in one-rescuer CPR?

    _____

11. Where do you push on the chest? _____

12. Do you pause between breaths in one-rescuer CPR? _____

REVIEW ANSWERS

Unit I

1. The phrase that will help you to remember the first steps for an unconscious person is "A Quick Check."

2. "A Quick Check" means:

   A = Airway: Tip head and check breathing.
   Quick = 4 quick, full breaths.
   Check = Check pulse and breathing.

3. Give 4 quick breaths at first.

4. Give 4 quick and full breaths.

5. After you give the first breaths, check the pulse and breathing.

6. The rate of mouth-to-mouth breathing for an adult is one breath every 5 seconds.

7. You might use mouth-to-nose breathing if your mouth is too small to make a seal or if the victim's mouth is injured.

8. You would try to give breaths without tipping the head (by jutting or thrusting the jaw) if the victim's neck or back is injured.

Unit 2

9. Give 80 compressions per minute in one-rescuer CPR.

10. The pattern of breaths and compressions in one-rescuer CPR is 2 breaths and 15 compressions.

11. Push on the lower half of the sternum for compressions.

12. No, give two breaths without a pause in one-rescuer CPR.

FINAL TEST
Form A

Do not take this test until you have completed all checkouts and Unit 3, Review.

Take this test in class with instructor supervision. Follow any special procedures your instructor has set up. Mark only one answer to each question. Please do not look back at the workbook while you take the test.

Your instructor may give you Test Form B to use instead of Form A. Form B covers the same basic material.

Unit I

1. Fill in the first steps for an unconscious person.

_____ = _____

_____ = _____

_____ = _____

2. What is the best way to find out if a person has stopped breathing?

[ ] a. Check the pulse.
[ ] b. Check the pupils of the eyes.
[ ] c. Look at the chest; listen and feel for air coming out of the mouth.

3. The 4 quick breaths for an adult should be

[ ] a. small, gentle breaths.
[ ] b. large, full breaths.

4. In caring for a victim of a violent accident, it is probably better to

[ ] a. check for breathing before you move the victim at all.
[ ] b. position the victim on the back for mouth-to-mouth breathing
or CPR immediately.

5. When rolling a victim onto the back for mouth-to-mouth breathing or
CPR, move the body

[ ] a. one part at a time; first the head, then the shoulders, then the legs.
[ ] b. in one motion; keep the body from twisting.

6. When you tip the head with the neck lift, the major force is applied with
the hand

[ ] a. on the forehead.
[ ] b. under the neck.

7. In mouth-to-mouth breathing, when you take a breath, turn your head
to look at the victim's

[ ] a. forehead.
[ ] b. chest.

8.   How long do you pause between each of the 4 quick breaths?

[ ]   a. About 3 seconds between each breath.
[ ]   b. Only long enough to get a breath.

9.   How often do you give breaths to an adult in mouth-to-mouth breathing after you give 4 quick breaths?

[ ]   a. Once every second.
[ ]   b. Once every 3 seconds.
[ ]   c. Once every 5 seconds.

10.   When you do the head tip—chin lift, place your fingertips under the

[ ]   a. bony part of the jaw near the chin.
[ ]   b. soft part of the throat near the chin.

11.   If the victim's mouth is injured, or your mouth is too small to give mouth-to-mouth breathing,

[ ]   a. wait for an ambulance equipped with breathing equipment.
[ ]   b. give mouth-to-~~mouth~~ breathing.
                      nose

12. You should push air out of the victim's stomach

[ ] a. whenever the stomach fills with air.
[ ] b. only when the stomach is bulging with air
         and you cannot inflate the lungs.

13. Which head tip method may work better for a person who has dentures?

[ ] a. Head tip—chin lift.
[ ] b. Head tip—neck lift.

14. If a person may have neck or back injuries, which is the safer way to open
    the airway?

[ ] a. Tip the head very gently, partway back.
[ ] b. Push the jaw forward from the corners.

Unit 2

15. How do you give chest compressions?

[ ] a. Smoothly and regularly.
[ ] b. With a quick jerk.

16. How far do you compress the chest of an adult?

[ ] a. At least 4 centimeters (1 1/2 to 2 inches).
[ ] b. At least 1 centimeter (1/4 to 1/2 inch).

17. For compressions to be effective, the victim must be on a

[ ] a. soft surface.
[ ] b. hard surface.

18. How do you find where to push on the chest?

[ ] a. Measure up one finger-width from the middle finger on the notch.
[ ] b. Push on the xiphoid.

19. How do you push on a victim's chest?

[ ] a. Straight down.
[ ] b. At an angle.

20. Pushing on the xiphoid is likely to

[ ] a. increase the amount of blood circulation.
[ ] b. cause internal injuries.

21. At what rate do you give chest compressions to an adult in one-rescuer CPR?

[ ] a. 40 per minute.
[ ] b. 60 per minute.
[ ] c. 80 per minute.
[ ] d. 100 per minute.

22.	In one-rescuer CPR, what is the pattern of compressions and breaths?

[ ]	a.	5 compressions, then one breath.
[ ]	b.	5 compressions, then 2 breaths.
[ ]	c.	15 compressions, then one breath.
[ ]	d.	15 compressions, then 2 breaths.

23.	How long do you check the pulse before deciding whether CPR is needed?

[ ]	a.	1–3 seconds.
[ ]	b.	3–5 seconds.
[ ]	c.	5–10 seconds.
[ ]	d.	10–20 seconds.

24. You are giving CPR and find that pulse and breathing start again. What should you do next?

[ ] a. Get the victim to a life-support unit.
[ ] b. Continue mouth-to-mouth breathing without chest compressions.
[ ] c. Continue chest compressions without mouth-to-mouth breathing.
[ ] d. Continue CPR.

25. CPR should be given until

[ ] a. you know that an ambulance is on the way.
[ ] b. other persons take over, or the heart starts to beat.